The management of epilepsy in dogs

Second Edition

Phyllis G Croft
OBE, PhD FRCVS

I

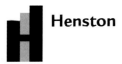

Henston

Henston

Produced in association with Vetoquinoi

Henston
A Division of Veterinary Business Development
Olympus House
Werrington Centre
Peterborough PE4 6NA
Telephone: +44 (0)1733 325522
Facsimile: +44 (0) 1733 325512
e-mail: henston@vetsonline.com

Designed and produced by Veterinary Business Development Ltd

ISBN 1 85054 097 7

First published 1984
Reprinted 1986, 1988
Second edition 1994
Third edition 2000

® 1999 Veterinary Business Development Ltd

Price £7.50

II

About the author

Phyllis Croft OBE, PhD FRCVS

Became interested in canine epilepsy in the 1930s when a succession of her family's Beagle puppies developed fits. In 1944 she was awarded a PhD for her thesis on mental disease; after qualifying MRCVS in 1950 she took up electro-encephalography as a means of studying epilepsy in animals, and received the Livesey Medal for work in this field. For the past thirty five years she has worked as a veterinary consultant for diseases of the brain, and in 1959 received a Fellowship for her thesis on this subject. She was invited to speak on epilepsy at the World Veterinary Congress in Greece in 1975. In 2000 was awarded the OBE by H.M. the Queen for services to animals and humanity.

III

Contents

Preface

This book is written in the hope that it may help all those who are interested in the problems associated with epilepsy in dogs. The successful treatment and management of animals with fits depends essentially on teamwork: on the specialised knowledge of the veterinarian, on the common sense and powers of observation of the owner, and on the interest and understanding of the breeder. Finally, any attempt at teamwork will be frustrated if the lines of communication are not good, and veterinary nurses are very important here.

The text has been kept as simple as possible and a glossary is provided – so that all the members of the team can understand and use it for the better management of animals with epilepsy. In addition, veterinary students who have reached the clinical years of their training should find it a useful supplement to their notes on the diseases of the nervous system.

Knowledge of epilepsy is an important point of contact between medical and veterinary practitioners methods of differential diagnosis and of treatment are comparable in human and veterinary medicine. Hence, epilepsy is one of the fields in which doctor and veterinary surgeon can usefully exchange experiences, and collaborate in research.

Epilepsy is known to occur in most of the species treated by veterinarians in general practice, but it is far more common in the dog than in any other species. This book is therefore based on epilepsy as seen in the dog, but where important differences occur in other species, these will be mentioned.

V

Introduction

Epilepsy was certainly described by the ancient Greeks and it may be that the rush of the Gadarene swine was an example of the condition. The term is derived from the Greek word meaning "to lay upon" or "to seize" and in ancient times the victim was believed to have been "seized" by angry gods; it was also thought that the patient's breath might infect others, and hence epileptics were generally shunned. Hippocrates was the first person to suggest a natural, rather than a demonic, aetiology for convulsions, but superstitions and folk-lore persisted until the late nineteenth century when the studies of Hughlings Jackson provided the basis for modern therapy and understanding. Since that time, electro-encephalography and, more recently, MRI scanning have paved the way for notable advances and, at the same time, education is slowly overcoming the irrational fears of those who have close contact with epileptic patients, both human and animal.

FEAR OF RABIES

In the veterinary sphere the situation is complicated by the genuine fear of rabies, but it must be remembered that only common conditions occur commonly, and in this country it is not really likely that a dog presenting with a fit has rabies. Nevertheless it is still important to remember that the veterinarian must pay due attention to the state of mind of the owner, as well as to the nervous system of the patient: the onset of a fit together with the distorted posture of the animal can cause an owner to suffer severe shock or hysteria, and it is not easy for the layman to accept that the patient is neither in pain, nor likely to die a horrible death in the near future. The alarm experienced by onlookers makes the veterinarian's work particularly difficult because his patient often appears quite normal by the time he sees it; he must, therefore, rely on others for a description of the attack, and panic and hysteria are not conducive to accurate observation. Hence, it is vital that the practitioner should know exactly which questions will give him the information he needs.

CO-OPERATION

Mutual trust and co-operation between the veterinary surgeon and his client are essential throughout the management of the case; the veterinary surgeon will probably need to rely on the observations of the owner to determine the optimum dose of anti-convulsant, and even the choice of drug may require the help of the client. Epilepsy is a field in which there is little opportunity for a "rule of thumb" approach but, on the other hand, there is great scope for teamwork between breeders, owners, clinicians and research workers.

Epilepsy is characterised by abnormal paroxysmal discharges in the brain which give rise to a chronically recurring loss of consciousness. Thus, epilepsy is a sign, not a disease. Any condition which damages the brain may cause epilepsy, and any congenital abnormality which leads to imperfect insulation, or hyperexcitability, of neurons may also give rise to it.

Apart from this multiple aetiology, the clinical manifestations also cover a wide range because they depend on the area of the brain affected, and on whether the abnormal activity remains localised, or spreads to involve the whole brain. Thus, it becomes obvious that to give a diagnosis of "epilepsy" when an animal presents with a fit, is doing little more that state the obvious; it gives no real information as to aetiology, therapy or prognosis, and leaves the client with no useful guidance as to the management of the patient in the future.

DIFFERENTIAL DIAGNOSIS

Cases of epilepsy can be successfully treated, but since there are many different causes, accurate differential diagnosis is an essential first stage in therapy. The co-operation of the owner as an observer is particularly important and, in return, the veterinarian must be prepared to inform and re-assure his client. If, on the other hand, a client is knowledgeable about the situation, the veterinary surgeon must be able to give advice about breeding plans, or at least be able to direct the client to a source of expert advice.

1 Aetiology

The causes of epilepsy can conveniently be divided into those deriving **wholly from the pathology of the brain or nervous system**, and those stemming originally from pathology of some other organ or system. First, however, it is important to be quite clear about the clinical entity described as a fit, since animals can have a variety of "attacks" or "queer turns" which should not be confused with fits.

Description of fit. Essential distinguishing features

A fit may be defined as an incident of very short duration, characterised by at least a few moments of unconsciousness, and by tonic and clonic stages; involuntary defaecation and urination may occur during the fit, and the animal is often ravenously hungry on recovery. The inter-ictal behaviour of the animal is normal, although in some animals there may be an "aura" for a few minutes prior to the onset of the fit itself. **Fits almost always occur when an animal is relaxed in its own home surroundings and, frequently, when the animal is asleep.**

The foregoing is a description of a typical fit in a dog and corresponds, roughly, to the Grand Mal convulsion of a human being with epilepsy. Many variations are seen, but the above is by far the most common. In the cat and the horse the common form of epilepsy is different; in these species the animal first runs wildly- round the house in the case of the cat, and straight through several fields in the case of a horse at grass. This can be very frightening for onlookers, particularly since horses will crash through fences and may reach a tarmac road and cause a traffic accident. This running phase can last for some minutes and is usually succeeded by collapse and a classical convulsion. **The essential features of an epileptic fit which distinguish it from most of the other attacks witnessed in animals are (a) that it occurs when the animal is relaxed and (b) that the animal is completely disconnected from its surroundings for, at least, part of the fit.**

Causes originating from the brain or nervous system

Some epileptogenic conditions are common in puppies, some in young dogs and others in dogs past middle-age, **so it is convenient to look at possible aetiologies with the age of the animal in mind.**

Trauma and anoxia

In the first place, there are various accidents which may occur at birth or immediately after; these do not necessarily give rise to fits until some weeks later and by that time the original mishap may have been forgotten. If the pup does not breathe immediately after birth, cerebral anoxia may occur and some part of the brain may be temporarily or permanently damaged; this may cause fits at the time, or later. Again, the pup may be damaged at birth by forceps or it may fall out of a whelping box, or be kicked out, or it may be dropped by a human unused to holding such a small lively object; any of these mishaps can produce a head injury which will eventually give rise to an epileptogenic focus in the brain. It is not unusual for a maiden bitch to be frightened by the birth of her first pup and run about with it before the umbilical cord has been broken, and this also can lead to a head injury and subsequent epilepsy.

Internal hydrocephalus: predisposition in some breeds

Another common cause of fits in young puppies is congenital internal hydrocephalus; this is most commonly seen in breeds with domed skulls such as the chihuahua, toy poodle or King Charles spaniel, but it can occur in any breed; it may be accompanied by an open fontanelle, but this is not necessarily so, and there may likewise be an open fontanelle without any clinical abnormality. Internal hydrocephalus may present as fits, but it may also give rise to a variety of other clinical symptoms. It has been suggested that there is a hereditary tendency to this condition in certain breeding lines in some breeds, but rigid proof for this is lacking, and it is probably better, therefore, to regard it as an anatomical weakness in certain breeds.

Effects of diet

The possible influence of diet on the causation of fits can best be considered while dealing with puppies, though it can be relevant at any age. Owners frequently suggest that some small change in diet may have caused a fit but, in practice, nowadays this is rare; some fifty years ago dog biscuits contained a bleaching agent, agene, and consumption of such biscuits undoubtedly caused fits in dogs. Many owners have some vague memory of this, or have heard others talk of it, and are prepared to think that similar biscuits are still on the market. In fact, agene as a bleach for flour has been forbidden by law for many years. Occasionally, however, a batch of food sold in a pet shop does have some deleterious substance in it, usually intended as a preservative, and this may cause fits, but in such cases there is usually an "epidemic" of fits in a particular area, and the veterinary surgeon will know about this, and should be able to trace the source of the trouble fairly easily.

There is slightly more risk of diet-induced fits in cats, partly because they frequently have a diet containing only one or two different items in it, and partly because a fish diet can lead to a high concentration of the enzyme which destroys vitamin B in the blood, and adequate levels of vitamin B are essential for the proper functioning of the central nervous system.

Poisons

Poisoning can occur in animals of any age but the omnivorous habits of puppies do lead to special problems in dogs of three to nine months of age. Fits can occur as a sequel to the ingestion of a variety of substances but, in practice, the convulsant most commonly consumed by animals is metaldehyde in the form of slug bait. Other toxic substances produce a variety of signs some related to the alimentary tract and some to the nervous system but, in general, inhibition in the form of paralysis is more common than excitation. The widespread use of poisons, such as rat poisons and rodenticides, based on warfarin means that this substance must always be considered in cases of unknown aetiology: haemorrhages can occur in any part of the affected animal and instances are on record of patients which presented with fits, and were found at post-mortem examination to have large haematomata in the cerebro-vascular system. It is also as well to remember that puppies are often dosed with vermifuges by their owners, and unexpected reactions can occur in individual animals.

Canine distemper. Vaccine reactions

Canine distemper must still be included among the possible causes of fits in young dogs. The disease is not difficult to diagnose when nasal discharge and conjunctivitis occur in the unvaccinated dog, but the effects on the central nervous system may not be apparent until a month or two after apparent recovery. If the pup has changed owners (and veterinary surgeons) between the initial illness and the occurrence of the first fit, it may not be easy to trace the connection. Even in the young vaccinated dog it is possible to see fits which are due to viral or bacterial encephalitis. There is also the occasional animal which reacts abnormally to vaccination and, though it is almost impossible to prove that the damage to the nervous system is due to vaccine, it does sometimes seem that this is the most likely explanation.

Causes of encephalitis

When encephalitis is suspected, it is not usually possible to determine the nature of the causative organism but, undoubtedly, bacterial, viral and protozoal infections do occur. Moreover, the infection can be blood-borne from a remote infected area (eg anal glands), or it can arise as a spread from a contiguous area (eg nasal sinus or inner ear).

Primary epilepsy. Fit threshold

In the young adult dog, there are other more likely causes of fits; the commonest of these is primary epilepsy, also known as asymptomatic or idiopathic epilepsy. This is a condition which, as its name implies, has no pathology and the affected animal shows no signs of inter-ictal malaise; the individual concerned simply has a lower fit threshold than normal and so stimuli which would not affect other individuals, trigger convulsions in the particular animal. Much work has been done on the possible hereditary aspect of this condition in different species, but our knowledge is still very incomplete.

Fits in older dogs. Tumours and cerebro-vascular disease

From middle-age onwards the likelihood of a brain tumour causing epilepsy becomes more probable and in this age-range the possibility of cerebro-vascular disease and of cerebro-vascular accidents, must also be borne in mind. Differential diagnosis between a tumour and a cerebro-vascular accident is important since the prognosis for a cerebro-vascular accident is much more hopeful than that for a brain tumour.

Obviously most of these causes can be found in animals of any age, but the foregoing gives a rough guide; it is based on figures taken from 20,000 cases in the author's practice.

Extra-cerebal Causes

Physiology of brain cells

Brain cells, in order to function effectively, require a particular biochemical milieu, an adequate blood supply, a suitable oxygen-carbon dioxide balance and a sufficient, but not excessive, stream of incoming electrical signals from the peripheral nervous system. Any illness which affects any of these factors may give rise to fits, and it is important to recognise and treat the underlying cause as well as the fits.

Teething, parasitic worms and strychnine

Again, considering first the puppy, excessive stimulation of the peripheral nervous system may occur during teething, or if the animal is infested with parasitic worms, and this stimulation can trigger a form of convulsion. Strychnine poisoning should perhaps be mentioned here, too; the effect is essentially on the spinal cord but this leads to a spasm of the respiratory muscles, and so the initial spinal convulsion soon spreads to involve the brain through cerebral anoxia.

Toxaemia

The activity of the liver and kidneys is vital in maintaining the stability of the biochemical milieu and, where either of these systems is faulty, epilepsy may occur as a complication of toxaemia. This, of course, is more likely to be seen in the adult or ageing animal. The undiagnosed diabetic or the animal with islet-cell tumour of the pancreas falls into a similar category and although the presenting sign then is usually coma, hypo- or hyper-glycaemia can cause convulsions.

Hyperventilation

Overbreathing, which decreases the carbon dioxide pressure of the blood, is routinely used to precipitate fits in susceptible human beings, and it can also be so used in dogs; this fact can be significant when an animal is being artificially ventilated while under a general anaesthetic. Increased pressure of carbon dioxide can also trigger fits, and this has been known to occur during long car journeys in cold weather when ventilation is at a minimum. A similar situation can occur in an aeroplane.

Heart disease

Finally, among the extra-cerebral causes of fits, the heart must be mentioned. It should be possible to distinguish a faint from a fit by asking a witness the right questions; a slight cardiac defect may, however, first become apparent when the animal has a true fit. This occurs because the cerebro-vascular supply is defective: brain cells are more sensitive to an impaired blood supply than those in any other part of the body, so slight cardiac defects may well affect cerebral function in the first instance. It is, in fact, quite common for a dog which has had a cerebro-vascular accident, to show abnormalities on the electrocardiogram although, up to that time, there has been nothing to suggest heart disease.

5

There is also the rare situation when an animal survives a brief cardiac arrest (electric shock, anaesthetic accident, etc); this can lead to anoxic brain damage and eventually to fits.

2 Clinical conditions accompanied by fits

A fit is a sign and while, in some patients, it may be one of a group of signs making diagnosis easy, in many cases it is the only presenting sign, and differential diagnosis is difficult. Successful therapy does depend, in the first instance, on accurate diagnosis, so an attempt must be made. The first step in diagnosis depends on a good knowledge of the various conditions in which fits can occur. In this chapter the more common conditions involving fits are described; they are arranged with the common conditions at the beginning and the rarer ones at the end.

Primary Epilepsy

This condition is also known as idiopathic or asymptomatic epilepsy; these names explain its essential nature, for the fits have no obvious cause and post-mortem examination reveals no lesion in the brain or skull. Primary epilepsy is a functional disorder in which the affected animal's brain cells occasionally respond in an exaggerated manner to a normal stimulus. Any animal is capable of a convulsion, given an adequate stimulus, but the epileptic animal convulses much more readily than the majority of its species: its fit threshold is lower.

Precipitating factors

Precipitating factors include sleep, oestrus, water-loading and pyrexia. It is possible that heredity plays some part in determining an animal's fit threshold, but further research is necessary before the subject is fully understood. The term "idiopathic epilepsy" implies that the condition is an integral part of the animal's make-up, and this suggests that no treatment is likely to provide a radical cure; on the other hand, for the same reason, primary epilepsy does not itself become more serious during a dog's lifetime: many animals live a normal lifespan with primary epilepsy, and finally die from some other cause.

Typical signs. Effect on work and intelligence

Convulsions normally occur when an animal is relaxed or asleep; this means that the management of an epileptic animal need not involve any reduction in activity – in fact, police dogs and guide dogs for the blind can continue to work while suffering from primary epilepsy, and there is at least one race horse which has continued to race after a diagnosis of primary epilepsy. This also means that affected dogs are unlikely to have a fit while in the show-ring; moreover, where dogs sleep outside in kennels, it is quite possible for owners to be unaware that they possess dogs with primary epilepsy.

This situation can lead to great confusion: a breeder may sell a dog which he genuinely believes to be healthy, because any fits which it has, occur when it is in its kennel; if the new owner then keeps the dog indoors at night – maybe even in his own bedroom – then the fits will be observed. Clients do, in fact, find it very difficult to realise that fits occur in relaxation or sleep, although their own observations confirm the fact; they still try to relate the fit to some excitement or exertion that took place earlier. They also fear that intelligence will deteriorate, but this does not happen; guide dogs with primary epilepsy can continue to work.

Pattern of fit

The first fit which an owner observes usually occurs when a dog is between one and three years of age; since it commonly happens when the dog is asleep, the owner's attention may only be aroused in the middle of the fit when, for instance, the dog's feet are knocking repeatedly against the wall, or a piece of furniture. This is, in fact, the clonic phase of the fit and it has normally been preceded by a tonic phase, each of these phases lasting anything from a few seconds to a few minutes. The clonic stage gradually subsides and, after a short interval, the dog starts struggling to get on its feet. Respiratory and cardiac rhythms are severely disorganised by the tonic/clonic phases and, if an owner or veterinary surgeon examines the patient immediately after, he may mistakenly assume that a heart attack has taken place: in fact, the abnormal pulse and respiration is a **consequence** of the cerebral activity, not the cause of it.

A dog is totally unaware of its surroundings during a fit and, as it recovers, there is often a stage in which it is on its feet but does not yet recognise the people around it. During this period there is a danger that a normally gentle animal may bite someone, and it is important that the owner appreciates this, both for his own sake and for the sake of children or visitors who may not be familiar with the situation.

Recovery stage

The recovery stage of a fit is very variable, both in pattern and duration. At best, the animal may return to normality within a minute or two; in this case, it just suddenly looks round quite naturally, comes over to its owner for a pat, and then trots off as if nothing had happened. On the other hand, it may be an hour or so before the dog seems to be itself again; it will pace up and down, and round and round, compulsively for many minutes and it is not possible to "get through" to it at this time.

Sight seems to be the last sense to return fully, and so the animal blunders about, knocking into furniture, walls, bowls of water etc. This often leads the owner to report that the dog is going blind; it is as well for the veterinarian to be aware of this possible train of events and to be prepared to explain them to the owner if indeed the dog's sight appears to be normal when he examines it, after the fit.

If during this confused post-ictal stage, the dog comes across any food (perhaps the remains of an earlier meal), it often gulps it down ravenously, again without really seeming to be conscious of what it is doing. This stage can be very distressing to the owner, and there is little he can do to shorten or alter it. It usually ends with the animal tiring and lying down to sleep. The sleep seems natural, and when the animal wakes it is, in all respects, normal. The veterinary surgeon seldom sees it before this so he is very dependent on the owner for information as to the nature of the attack.

Occurrence and frequency. Linkage with oestrous cycle

Fits occur sporadically in primary epilepsy and it is seldom possible to find any temporal pattern for them; this makes it difficult to assess the value of any treatment, and often leads to owners worrying unnecessarily when, perhaps, a dog has two fits in twenty four hours after being fit-free for a month or two. If the patient is a bitch, it is worth noting if the fit frequency is related to the oestrous cycle; if a connection really does exist, it is an indication for spaying, or possibly hormonal control of oestrus.

Status epilepticus

Occasionally a dog with primary epilepsy goes into status epilepticus and has one fit after another for many hours; this is an emergency and the dog must be hospitalised and anaesthetised if it is to survive. Treatment is worthwhile because it is quite possible for a dog to live many years after such an incident, provided that the duration of status is not too long before anaesthesia is achieved.

Significance of increasing frequency of fits

Primary epilepsy does not become more serious with age; if a dog's fits are really becoming more frequent, it is quite possible that the dog has some sub-clinical condition unconnected with the nervous system (eg interstitial nephritis), because any departure from full health can lower the fit threshold. If the problem can be identified and treated successfully, then the fit threshold should return to its earlier level.

Temperament

Owners often worry about the possibility of a dog with primary epilepsy showing a change of temperament and becoming vicious: there is no evidence to show that this ever happens, although, as stated earlier, it is always unwise to approach a dog before it has become fully re-orientated after a fit. Occasionally a dog goes into a fit in a dangerous situation – on the edge of a pond, or at the top of a flight of stairs – and in such cases it is best to throw a coat or blanket over the patient and push or pull it to safety.

Television

In the medical world, theories circulate from time to time about the precipitation of fits by flickering television screens; this, in turn, leads to dog-owners suggesting that their dogs have fits because they lie near or under the TV set. There is no evidence to suggest that flickering light can precipitate fits in animals, and the reason for the dog having a fit while under the TV is simply that this is the place in which the animal usually relaxes or sleeps, and there is also the fact that the owner is likely to see any fits which occur in these circumstances.

Tonic epilepsy

The foregoing is a description of the form of epilepsy seen in the vast majority of dogs and it corresponds with the Grand Mal attack seen in human epilepsy; variants do, however, occur and most of the forms described in human medicine are occasionally recorded in dogs. The only variant which occurs with sufficient frequency to warrant description is that known as "tonic epilepsy", the tonic referring to the state of the musculature.

The usual description of this attack is simply that the dog suddenly stands still and no longer responds to the owner's voice; the whole incident is over in a minute or two but, unlike the Grand Mal convulsion, it does take place while the dog is in active movement, and can constitute a problem for a working guide dog. These attacks occur more often in Labradors than in any other breed and there is some evidence to suggest that the condition is common in certain lines within the breed. This form of attack is not frightening to the onlooker and in many cases it may not be reported to the veterinarian, but it is useful to know that it is a variant of epilepsy and can, if necessary, be treated with anti-convulsants; this fact, together with electroencephalographic recordings made during attacks, confirm that the condition should be considered as primary epilepsy.

Internal Hydrocephalus

Definition

Internal hydrocephalus is a condition in which there is excess fluid in the skull cavity and, hence, undue pressure on one or more parts of the brain. It is one of the most common congenital abnormalities in the dog and can be found in most of the other species with which the veterinarian comes into contact. The severity of the condition varies, from that in which clinical signs are barely apparent, to that in which euthanasia is the only reasonable solution; and since a patient may proceed from one state to the other in a fairly short time, diagnosis and treatment are important.

Aetiology

Hydrocephalus can be congenital or acquired; therapy is similar for the two conditions but the prognosis for the acquired condition is better, provided that the underlying cause can be treated successfully.

Breed tendencies

Some dog-breeders have suspected a hereditary factor in the aetiology, but it is doubtful if this can be substantiated. Certainly, some breeds of dog are prone to hydrocephalus because of the domed nature of their skulls; among these are the following: chihuahuas, papillons, griffons, King Charles spaniels and bulldogs. In these breeds certain familial tendencies to hydrocephalus can often be traced, but this is the most that can be stated with certainty.

Clinical picture

The clinical picture in the congenital case presents certain features which are not fully understood; a puppy may appear normal up to the age of, perhaps, eight weeks and then suddenly start to have fits and become ataxic and, within a few days, be totally paralysed. On post-mortem examination, the brain of such a puppy is often found to consist of only a few millimetres of brain tissue covering greatly dilated ventricles; it is obvious that the brain must have been very abnormal, anatomically, for some time, and it seems strange that the patient's illness only became apparent a day or two before death.

Causes of acquired condition

Acquired hydrocephalus can occur in any breed but, again, it is seen more commonly in breeds with rounded skulls. It can arise whenever there is cerebral oedema, or if there is some disturbance in the water balance of the patient. In practice, encephalitis and head injury are the most common causes of acquired internal hydrocephalus.

Diagnosis. Need for early therapy

Diagnosis of the congenital condition is not always easy. If the signs suggest involvement of the central nervous system and the superior fontanelle is open, internal hydrocephalus is probable; if there is no open fontanelle, but the puppy has a domed skull, then hydrocephalus should certainly be considered. The initial signs may occur at any time between birth and about nine months of age, and they take one or more of a variety of forms: there may be fits, attacks of some other type, locomotor disturbance, blindness, howling or vomiting. It is possible to confirm diagnosis by electro-encephalography, but since this will take some time, it is advisable to start therapy in the form of a diuretic whenever hydrocephalus is suspected; immediate treatment is desirable because, if hydrocephalus is present, permanent brain damage will result from pressure atrophy, and the extent of area affected will be related to the duration of the pressure.

Meningitis

Signs

The incidence of meningitis has been greatly reduced by routine vaccination against canine distemper, but the condition is still seen in puppies and young dogs. It is a dangerous illness because the onset is normally rapid and within 24 hours of the first signs of malaise, the dog may be dangerously ill and in need of expert treatment if it is to survive. Fits may occur, but they are not always present; the dog loses its appetite and behaves in a bizarre manner often cringing in dark places and crying without obvious cause; the cry is diagnostic of meningitis and once it has been heard, its recognition forms a very useful diagnostic clue. Interestingly enough, a comparable "meningitis cry" is recognised in human medicine. The other characteristics of the canine condition are pyrexia, often up to 105°F or even 106°F (40°C – 41°C), and hypersensitivity to touch in the cervical and occipital areas; this last feature suggests that the animal may have pain corresponding to the headache of a human being.

Prognosis and transmissibility

If a dog survives beyond the first two or three days of the illness, it has a good chance of recovering; there is, however, always the possibility of fits recurring at some later date – even three months after the acute phase has passed. These fits can usually be controlled reasonably well with an anti-convulsant, and they tend to become less severe as time passes. The condition does not seem to be highly contagious; probably, by the time the organisms are affecting the brain, they are not readily passed to the external atmosphere. There is likewise no evidence to suggest that the condition is transmissible to human beings.

Aetiology

The causal organism cannot normally be identified; it may be viral, bacterial or protozoal but the response to antibiotics suggests that it is often bacterial.

The organism can be blood-borne from an infective focus elsewhere in the body (in one animal an infected anal gland was the original focus), or spread can occur from an adjacent area such as sinus, ear or throat. In any case, it is wise to check for the presence of sites of chronic infection because it is very disappointing for all concerned to see a patient recover from severe meningitis and then relapse, and this can easily happen if there is a continuing source of infection. Relapses do also occur if the infection is due to a mixed population of bacteria, some of which are not sensitive to the antibiotic used. Such cases present a problem but sometimes they can be resolved by intelligent use of an alternative antibiotic.

Encephalitis

Signs, causes and prognosis

Meningitis obviously may spread to become meningo-encephalitis and the prognosis for this is grave. Encephalitis alone is most often seen as a relatively mild chronic condition not involving the meninges. Signs vary with the particular area of the brain involved, but it is quite common for this condition to present with fits. The cause may be infective or toxic, and the toxic form may be due to ingestion of poison, or to an internal toxaemia, possibly associated with poor liver or kidney function. The infective type is more common in young animals, whilst the toxaemic form is usually associated with older animals.

Head Injury

Causes

The most common cause of head injuries in small animals is road traffic accidents, but cats and dogs also get kicked by human beings and by horses, horses kick each other, children drop puppies on their heads, golfers hit dogs with golf balls, young active dogs run into tree-trunks – the list is endless. Owners sometimes report that a dog has fallen downstairs and subsequently started a fit; whilst this may be true in some cases, it is also possible that the dog had its first fit at the top of the stairs, and the fall was really just a consequence of the start of the fit.

Onset and signs

If fits occur as a result of a head injury, there is usually an interval of weeks or months between the accident and the first fit: this is because the fit is the result of the formation of scar tissue in the brain. This scar tissue forms an irritative focus in the brain and gives rise to **secondary** (or symptomatic) epilepsy. The signs seen at the time may be minimal – just a moment of unconsciousness, perhaps – and there may be no obvious skin lesion on the head, and certainly radiography may not reveal any skull fracture.

History diagnosis

Owners frequently do not realise that there can be a long gap between the accident and the first fit, and when attempting to establish a differential diagnosis, it is important to make this clear, so that an accurate history can be obtained.

Site of lesions

It is worth noting, for the few occasions when the point of impact on the skull is known, that the brain damage is often found on the opposite side. This phenomenon is also seen in human medicine where it is known as a "contre-coup" lesion; the blow on the skull causes the brain to travel across the skull cavity so that the lesion arises as it hits the far side.

Cerebro-vascular Disease

13

Causes. Pathology

Cerebro-vascular disease is seen in most vertebrates and is commonly associated with ageing; it gives rise to a variety of signs according to the particular area of the brain affected. The severity of the condition, speed of onset of signs, and prognosis depend largely on whether or not a cerebral haemorrhage has taken place. Cerebro-vascular disease can also arise from ingestion of toxic substances, and as a complication of encephalitis or meningitis; in these infections, microscopy often reveals "cuffing" of cerebral blood vessels and, when this has happened, the walls of the blood vessels are weakened and predisposed to provide sites for cerebro-vascular accidents.

Signs

Two separate clinical entities must be considered: chronic cerebro-vascular disease and an acute cerebro-vascular accident. The former may give rise to the latter but does not necessarily do so. In elderly patients, fits may be the only sign of cerebro-vascular disease; they occur with ever-increasing frequency, and tend to last longer as the months go by.

Treatment and prognosis

Some control is possible with anti-convulsants, but the prognosis is not good and, sooner or later, euthanasia is inevitable. If the disease is diagnosed at an early stage, further deterioration can be arrested by appropriate medication; cats respond particularly well and may live many years without further deterioration.

Cerebro-vascular Accident (CVA)

Distinguishing features of cerebro-vascular accident, treatment and prognosis

A cerebro-vascular accident is quite different in that it is characterised by sudden onset; fits are not the usual presenting sign, but occasionally an animal does present with a series of violent fits, with only a few minutes between each convulsion. If this situation persists for more than 15 – 20 minutes, the veterinary surgeon must give the animal a general anaesthetic, since repeated convulsion will affect respiration, and then the brain may sustain permanent damage from anoxia. Hopefully, if the animal can be kept from returning to full consciousness for 24 hours, it will not convulse further and there may then be no permanent brain damage. There is always the risk that further cerebro-vascular accidents will occur in the future because the factors which facilitated the original accident are likely still to be present.

Cardiac function and haemoglobin levels.
Rickets

Whenever a defect in cerebral circulation is suspected, cardiac function should be checked, and haemoglobin level, because these can cause similar signs to cerebro-vascular disease, or can aggravate the signs of mild cerebro-vascular disease. If similar signs are seen in a young animal, the most likely cause is some abnormality of the cervical vertebrae, or of the skull, constricting an artery. Rickets can cause such malformations in the skull but these cases are rare at the present time.

Occurrence of minor cerebro-vascular accidents.
Prognosis

Dogs and cats often have a history of a series of small cerebro-vascular accidents with months, or even years, between them, and the owner does not seek veterinary advice because recovery is rapid. Eventually a major accident takes place, and then the history of several lesser incidents in the past is very helpful in establishing a differential diagnosis. The prognosis for cerebro-vascular accidents in animals is, in general, better than in human beings, and recovery from a first accident is often complete in a week or two. The only exception to this is when sight is involved; loss of sight is usually permanent.

Space-occupyinig Lesion

Causes

A space-occupying lesion can be an abscess, cyst, haematoma, neoplasm or foreign body but, in fact, the majority of cases seen are neoplastic. As in cerebro-vascular disease, fits are not the common presenting sign but they often occur at some stage of the illness.

Signs of neoplasia

The typical case of cerebral neoplasia is characterised by a variety of signs in the one patient; they may be locomotor, sensory, behavioural and convulsive, all varying somewhat from day to day, but gradually becoming more severe. An advanced case often shows atrophy of the temporal muscles before any generalised wasting occurs; cerebral neoplasia can be secondary to a primary mammary tumour, so it is always worth checking on the existence, past or present, of other tumours.

Pain

Owners are often concerned about the existence of pain in a dog with a space-occupying lesion when other symptoms are not too severe; advanced cases usually seek to press their heads against a wall and this must be interpreted as a sign of pain (comparable with a headache in a human being), but if the animal is not behaving in this way, and shows no other obvious signs of pain, it is reasonable to re-assure the owner as to the patient's comfort.

Treatment

Occasionally, if the lesion is circumscribed and located on the surface of the brain, surgery may be possible, but in most cases little can be done in the way of treatment, other than symptomatic relief. Corticosteroids, sometimes seem to produce an almost miraculous cure, but this is short-lived (a month or two at the most) and is usually followed by a relapse which proves fatal. The veterinary surgeon's role in a case of cerebral neoplasia requires great diplomacy, in that, sooner or later he will probably have to recommend euthanasia; he should not hesitate to call in a second opinion if this will enable the client to take the final decision with more confidence.

Summary

This chapter has dealt in some detail with the eight more common conditions involving fits in dogs. To form a quick method of reference to assist the busy veterinary surgeon the following table summarises the main aspects:

Condition	Major features	Distinguishing signs	Prognosis
Primary epilepsy	Fits.	Onset usually between 1 and 3 years old. Fits occur when dog is relaxed. No inter-ictal ill health.	Pharmaeological control usually possible.
Internal hydro-cephalus	Fits and/or ataxia and/or paralysis and/or abnormal behaviour.	Onset before 1 year old. Often associated with domed skull in small breeds.	Depends on severity and duration of un-treated condition.
Meningitis	Severe illness including fits.	Pyrexia. Photophobia. Occipital hypersensitivity. Unusual cry.	Fairly good if dog survives acute stage.
Encephalitis	Often chronic mild condition following infection elsewhere.	Fits can occur when dog is alert. Treatment difficult because relapses commonly occur.	Depends on nature of infec-ting organism.
Head injury	Interval between trauma and onset of fits is often several months	Accident at some time in history. Fits occur later without other signs of ill-health.	Good.
Cerebro-vascular disease	Fits. Attacks with muscular twitching. Various central nervous system defects depending on area of brain affected.	Progressive condition associated with ageing.	Poor.
Cerebro-vascular accident	Series of fits in quick succession. Lateralised paralysis.	Sudden onset of severe condition: torticollis often obvious. Gradual improvement in subsequent weeks.	Good, except when sight is affected.
Space-occupying lesion	Progressive illness with multiplicity of signs including fits.	Wasting. Head pressing. Compulsive pacing	Poor.

3 Differential diagnosis

Differential diagnosis of the cause of a fit is particularly difficult because the animal is usually normal by the time the veterinary surgeon sees it. So the practitioner relies largely on the owner's account and, whilst sometimes this may be very helpful, at other times it may be so vague and inaccurate as to be misleading. Fits do alarm people greatly, and in such conditions, scientific observation is impossible; on these occasions the veterinarian must exercise some skill and patience – in asking suitable questions so as to obtain the information he needs or, if that seems impossible, in encouraging the client to note useful points next time an attack occurs. Some owners have been able to make videos of their dogs' fits and these can be very useful. The sheets issued by Vétoquinol are helpful, in that they list a number of simple questions which the client should be able to answer; this helps him or her to feel part of a team working with the veterinarian to treat the animal correctly. This relationship is particularly valuable throughout the treatment of cases of epilepsy.

The following scheme summarises a plan of action which can be followed for differential diagnosis of the cause of an attack, which could be a fit, in a new patient.

Guide to differential diagnosis of fits in dogs

Cardiac
Occurs when active and awake. Vocalisation and retching common. Patient seeks and knows owner. Not spastic or distorted. Not disorientated. Duration very variable.

Cerebral
Occurs out of sleep or relaxation. Patient totally disorientated. Tonic and clonic stages. Duration of convulsions not greater than 3 min.

Internal hydrocephalus (congenital)
Patient less than 1 year old. Domed skull. Toy or small breed, usually, EEG or MRI very useful.

Encephalitis
Often chronic and mild. Usually extra-cerebral source/infection (ear, sinus, tooth, etc).

Cerebro-vascular disease
Patient past middle age. Short twitching attacks common. Progressive.

Space-occupying lesion
Patient past middle age. General progressive malaise. Assorted signs. Hypersensitive to CNS drugs. Head pressing. Temporal wasting.

Primary epilepsy
First attack between 1 and 3 years old. Inter-ictal health normal. Related animals may be affected.

Meningitis
Pyrexia. Hypersensitive in occipital/cervical area. Characteristic cry/howl. Usually severe and acute.

Cerebro-vascular accident
Very sudden onset. Torticollis and nystagmus. Laterality of signs.

Head injury
History of accident at some time – may be as much as two years previously.

Identification of system responsible for attack

History

The initial step in differential diagnosis of an attack is to establish whether or not it originates from the brain; the likely alternatives are the heart, the spinal cord or peripheral nervous system, or the biochemical balance of the blood. Information as to the circumstances in which the attack occurred, and the speed of onset, is the most useful.

Distinction between fit and cardiac attack

Fits caused by primary epilepsy, and the majority of the fits resulting from other causes, take place when the animal is relaxed or asleep, in its own familiar surroundings (home or car) and, as far as the observer is concerned, the onset is sudden and without vocalisation. Attacks of cardiac origin often occur when an animal is excited or frightened or has suddenly exerted itself (e.g. leapt up from sleep when doorbell or telephone bell has rung). The onset is not as sudden as that of a fit and the animal often cries as the attack starts or it may attempt to be sick; the cardiac attack does not have the tonic and clonic stages seen in a Grand Mal convulsion, and the patient does not lose touch with its surroundings – that is, it still shows response to its owner by eye movements, or by struggling to rise. By contrast, the animal that is having a fit is totally disconnected from its environment, and out of touch with its human attendants.

Almost all owners make some attempt to control or comfort their animals in heart attacks and in fits, and it is usually possible to discover from them whether or not the animal made an attempt to respond; this is probably the most useful single criterion for differentiating between attacks of cardiac and cerebral origin. Another small point that may be useful is to discover whether the animal seemed to go down on its **fore**legs first (cardiac attack), or to have difficulty in regaining use of its **hind**quarters after the attack (cerebral attack).

Detailed observations and common errors

More skilled observations, such as the colour of the tongue and mucous membranes, the nature of the pulse and respiration, may be possible if the owner has seen several attacks and is sufficiently clinically-minded. Such observations can, however, be misleading, in that the muscular contractions of a fit disorganise cardiac and respiratory rhythms, and for several minutes after a fit the pulse and respiration may be grossly abnormal; an owner may observe this state and tell the veterinary surgeon with confidence that his animal has had a "heart attack".

Fits and other attacks originating in the peripheral nervous system

Assuming that attacks of cardiac origin have been excluded, the veterinarian is now faced with deciding whether the attack originated in the brain or in some other part of the nervous system. Teething and internal parasites can excite the peripheral nervous system and give rise to attacks which could be confused with fits of cerebral origin: the age of the patient gives some clue, and it is not difficult to establish the presence or absence of the stimulus, if the age seems appropriate. Again, it is important to get a good description from the owner, because sometimes individual idiosyncrasies, such as turning round several times before defaecating, or twitching in sleep, are interpreted as "fits", particularly if the clients have not owned a dog before. Specific poisons can affect the peripheral nervous system but, in practice, this rarely leads to fits – some degree of paralysis is more common.

Strychnine poisoning

Attacks arising from the spinal nervous system are seen in cases of strychnine poisoning; in such cases the convulsion is precipitated by sudden sounds and the animal does not lose consciousness until asphyxia supervenes. Also, there is no clonic and tonic stage in the strychnine attack. The majority of other conditions affecting the spinal cord are degenerative and lead to paralysis rather than excitation, and, again, do not involve loss of consciousness or distortion.

Differential diagnosis of attacks arising from the brain (fits)

Assuming now that attacks arising from the cardio-vascular system and from peripheral and spinal nervous systems have been ruled out, it is necessary to differentiate between the many conditions that can affect the brain so as to give rise to a fit.

Information from the owner

Hopefully the owner, or someone who has seen the fit and knows the animal, will be present, and from their description the veterinarian is reasonably satisfied that the attack was a Grand Mal type of convulsion.

Genetic and peri-natal factors

Then it is advisable to review the animal's history, and to start with anything that is known about the patient's antecedents; if primary epilepsy has been diagnosed in any of these, this is a useful pointer but it is important not to jump to conclusions without a full investigation. It is useful to know if birth was normal or assisted; there is always a risk that in an assisted birth the young animal will have sustained a period of cerebral anoxia, and this can lead to permanent brain damage. There is also the point that assistance may have been necessary because an animal had a very domed skull and this could suggest the presence of internal hydrocephalus.

Vaccination status.

Head injuries

The vaccination history of the animal should be ascertained, and the possibility of any post-natal accident which might have led to a head injury. Owners often forget accidents that happened a year or more earlier, and they tend to think that if there was no obvious skin lesion in the head region, there was no possibility of a head injury. The veterinary surgeon also needs to be aware that someone, perhaps a child visitor, might have dropped a puppy on its head and then been too frightened to report the matter to a "grown-up".

Body tumours

The existence of tumours of any other part of the body should also be ascertained, or any earlier operations to remove "lumps"; the layman does not always connect a "little lump on the milk gland" with the possibility of a secondary tumour in the skull, particularly if he was assured at the time that the tumour was benign and had been satisfactorily removed.

Significance of frequency of fits

If the animal has had a number of fits, it is helpful to examine the dates to see if there is any pattern to them, suggesting some precipitating factor, or whether they are entirely sporadic; on the other hand, the fits may be becoming noticeably more frequent, suggesting a progressive condition rather than primary epilepsy. If the patient is female, it is worth investigating whether or not there is any correspondence between the oestrous cycle, and the fit frequency; this correspondence is apparent in quite a large proportion of the cases of primary epilepsy occurring in bitches and it can be a pointer to treatment .

Other signs of illness

It is also helpful to find out if the owner has noticed any signs of general malaise – unwillingness to go for walks, changes in appetite or thirst, loss of weight, dullness or actual loss of coat, loss of house-training, localised pain, etc.

Clinical examination by veterinary surgeon

When the practitioner has gained all the information he can from the owner and others associated with the general care of the patient, he must make his own examination. The following are some of the points which may help him to reach a correct diagnosis as to the cause of the fits.

Breed

Breeds of dog with small domed skulls (eg chihuahua, toy poodle, King Charles spaniel) are likely to suffer from internal hydrocephalus, both as a congenital abnormality, and as an acquired complication of other brain conditions such as head injuries. Heredity is known to play a part in the causation of primary epilepsy in a number of breeds and active research is in progress in this field. Boxers and labradors are among the breeds most likely to suffer from tumours.

Fits

Fits caused by irritation from intestinal parasites, and to emerging teeth are only likely to occur in puppies. Poisoning caused by ingestion of toys, pens etc is always a possibility in puppies. Head injuries can arise when a lively puppy is dropped or when a bitch pushes a pup out of a raised whelping-box. Encephalitis can occur as a complication of vaccination and, in any case, is more likely to occur in a young animal which has not yet developed a broad general immunity.

The first fit of primary epilepsy is usually seen when the dog is between one and three years of age. Cerebro-vascular accidents occur in dogs from middle-age onwards and in cats, at any age. Brain tumours mainly occur from middle-age onwards.

If the animal's health appears to be completely normal, both in the eyes of the owner and the veterinarian, it is very likely that the fits are due to primary epilepsy. Recent, or present, pyrexia, even of short duration is suggestive of encephalitis or, if it is severe and persistent, of meningitis. Any source of infection in the head and neck region (ears, tonsils etc), or the presence of enlarged glands in that region, points to the possibility of encephalitis. A choreic twitch commonly occurs as a result of an earlier attack of encephalitis and decreases with time.

General clinical picture

Unequal pupils, or any unilateral facial feature, including torticollis, is usually associated with a cerebro-vascular accident, or occasionally with a space-occupying lesion. Photophobia accompanied by pain in the occipital region and pyrexia are almost diagnostic of meningitis, particularly if there is also a "meningitis cry". Prolonged head-pressing into a wall or furniture is pathognomonic of a space-occupying lesion.

Specialised investigations

If the foregoing has not established a diagnosis, one or more specialised investigations may help. These include haematology, blood biochemistry and urinalysis, faecal examination, cerebro-spinal fluid analysis, ophthalmology, radiography, magnetic resonance imaging, electro-cardiography and electro-encephalography. If any of these is contemplated, it is advisable to contact the consultant concerned in advance and find out if any special conditions must be fulfilled regarding the patient or the specimen; if, for instance, the patient is having medication, it may be necessary to withdraw this before the test is carried out. The cost and preferred method of payment should also be ascertained; it is embarrassing for the owner to find that he is expected to pay the consultant at the time of examination, when he has supposed that he will be billed through his own veterinary surgeon later on. The approximate waiting time before a result can be expected is also important so that the owner is not disappointed by anticipating an "on-the-spot" result, when in fact he is going to have to wait some days.

If the owner is taking his animal to a consultant without his own veterinarian being present, it is essential that the practitioner writes a letter of referral, giving the history of the case and the treatment up to the time of consultation and any other details that may be useful, such as the fact that the client is a breeder, or needs the animal for working and is not interested in keeping it if it will not be able to work in the future. The practitioner should also ascertain whether general anaesthesia will be necessary and advise the owner accordingly. Even if the specialised examination is as objective as a blood count, it is still advisable to send details of history and treatment, because the significance of the report can almost always be amplified if the specialist has these details; this applies equally, whether the specialist is a veterinary surgeon or not.

Haematology

A differential white cell count may suggest the presence of an infection, but it is important to remember that a normal blood picture does not preclude the existence of encephalitis, any more than a normal temperature does; Lymphocytic leukaemia may also be brought to light from this examination. Prothrombin time may reveal ingestion of warfarin or a similar poison, and it may also give some guide as to the existence of a cerebro-vascular accident.

Blood biochemistry

Abnormal blood sugar may suggest that the "fits" are, in fact, hypoglycaemic attacks; serum calcium may be significant if the attacks have occurred during lactation. Liver function tests or blood urea nitrogen may reveal a toxic encephalopathy.

Urinalysis

Sometimes it is possible to obtain a urine sample more easily than a blood sample, and this may provide an initial pointer to diabetes mellitus or insipidus, or to kidney failure and subsequent toxaemia.

Faecal examination

The possibility of peripheral stimulation from gastro-intestinal parasites can be checked by faecal examination; again, diarrhoea may suggest poisoning, or an infection of the alimentary tract which might, later, appear as a blood-borne infection of the brain.

Cerebro-spinal fluid analysis

Specimens of cerebro-spinal fluid should only be taken by a veterinary surgeon who is familiar with the procedure, since the patient can easily be damaged, and, also, because it is important that the specimen is not contaminated with blood. As with haematological examinations, an abnormal result may give a definite pointer to a diagnosis, but a normal result does not preclude the presence of brain pathology.

Ophthalmoscopy

Ophthalmological examination can give indirect information about the state of the cerebro-vascular system, and about the optic nerve. Moreover, any defects seen may be present in one or both eyes, and this gives some help in assessing the extent of the pathology. The presence of a space-occupying lesion in the skull, or of cerebro-vascular disease may be inferred from ophthalmoscopy.

Radiography

The skull is a difficult area for radiography and, as with most of these specialised procedures, the results will only be useful in the hands of an expert. Sometimes it is possible to detect skull damage after a head injury and occasionally it is possible to discover a tumour with radiography. An abscess round the root of a tooth in the upper jaw, or in a sinus, might also be shown and could be significant as a focus of infection from which encephalitis could arise.

Magnetic Resonance Imaging

MRI is a non-invasive scanning procedure which gives a 3-dimentional picture of the brain showing its different parts. Space-occupying lesions and other abnormalities may be located by this procedure.

Electro-cardiography

It is desirable to have as much information about the heart as possible, primarily to determine whether the attack is cardiac or cerebral in origin and, secondarily, to discover whether the heart plays any significant part in the aetiology. It is possible, for instance, that a fit may be due to cerebro-vascular disease, but this condition is often aggravated by poor cardiac performance and, ideally, treatment for both the blood vessels and the heart should be instituted. Much information can be gained from auscultation, but electro-cardiography is a valuable supplement to the information provided by the stethoscope.

Electro-encephalography

Electro-encephalography procedure can be carried out with a minimum of disturbance in animals which can be handled easily and, in the hands of an experienced interpreter, gives a great deal of help in differential diagnosis of any cerebral condition. Interpretation is, however, difficult and it must be done by someone familiar with recordings from the species concerned; there is wide variation from one individual to another in normal records, and it is also easy to be misled by artefacts. Ideally, interpretation should be carried out by someone who is both clinician and electrophysiologist.

Scheme for consultations

A conclusive differential diagnosis may not be possible when a practitioner is first called to see an animal which has had some form of attack, but some advice must be given to the client, who is often greatly alarmed by what he has just seen. It should be possible, by asking the right questions, to make a well-informed guess. The outline scheme which follows has been found to work well in the hands of the author, but every practitioner will, no doubt, want to make his own modifications as his experience increases. The scheme, as described earlier in the chapter, has two parts: information from the owner, and clinical examination by the veterinarian.

(a) Information from the owner

QUESTION	COMMENTS
1. Was the present incident the first (as far as the owner knows)?	Treatment not usually necessary for isolated fit if animal appears healthy, but consider possibility of poisoning (see Question 13).
2. If so, how old is the dog now? If not, how old was the dog when the first incident occurred?	Internal hydrocephalus – common onset between one and six months. Primary epilepsy – common onset between one and six years. Tumour not common in young

dogs. Cerebro-vascular disease – not common in young dogs.

3. Have related, or "in contact", dogs shown the same signs?	Hereditary factor often present in primary epilepsy. Familial factor sometimes seen in internal hydrocephalus. Several dogs in one establishment affected, or ill in some way, suggests infection or poisoning.
4. Under what circumstances did attack occur? At home or out on a walk, relaxed or asleep or excited?	Primary epilepsy almost always occurs when dog is relaxed or asleep. Some heart conditions occur when a dog is suddenly excited – eg doorbell rings when dog is asleep.
5. What signs were shown? General description.	Make sure that description covers whole of attack – if it occurs at night, owner may only see latter part of it. It is vital to know if dog is aware of surroundings throughout the attack, but questions must be carefully worded, since many people equate unconsciousness with flaccidity, and do not realise that an animal in a state of tonic contraction, can be unconscious. Primary epilepsy of the Grand Mal type leads to a fit with a very definite pattern. Vocalisation at the beginning of an attack is usually a sign of a cardiac origin. Attacks lasting half an hour or more are usually cerebral, but not primary epilepsy.
6. How long did attack last?	Confirms or eliminates epilepsy.
7. How did dog behave after incident?	Ravenous consumption of food after the attack suggestive of cerebral rather than cardiac origin. If temperament changed post-ictally (to aggression), this must be considered in advising on management of future incidents.
8. Is dog healthy between attacks?	Normal with primary epilepsy.
9. Is there history of head injury at any time in dog's life (eg road traffic accident, kick by horse, blow from golfball, dropped as puppy, fall down stairs)?	Head injury can lead to secondary epilepsy, and there may be years between the accident and the first observed fit; the fact that the dog was "looked at" after the accident and pronounced all right does not preclude the possible development of secondary epilepsy later.

The management of epilepsy in dogs

10. Has the dog had any recent infections (eg canine distemper, "kennel cough", chronic otitis, infected upper teeth, anal adenitis etc)?

Any of these conditions could be associated with meningitis or encephalitis.

11. If a bitch, when was last oestrus, and is cycle regular?

Primary epilepsy can be oestrus-related and, if so, this may indicate the need for ovaro-hysterectomy or hormonal control. Irregular oestrous periods, or cessation of oestrus may indicate a tumour affecting the pituitary gland.

12. Has the dog undergone previous surgery?

Brain tumours are often secondary; information given to the owner to the effect that a previous tumour was not malignant is not always reliable. Aural resection suggests a focus of infection for meningitis; experience has also shown that ear infections are often associated with cerebral haemorrhages. Presence of aural haematoma might also be associated with cerebral haemorrhage.

13. Has the dog had access to poisons?

Pest control officers may assert that a substance is "harmless to pets" or has been put in an inaccessible position, but all such information is suspect. Slug pellets do not strike some owners as potentially dangerous.

(b) Clinical examination by veterinary surgeon

FACTOR

COMMENTS

1. Breed

Breeds with domed skulls have tendency to congenital internal hydrocephalus. Some breeds more susceptible to epilepsy than others – eg German shepherd dogs. Some breeds more likely to have tumours than others – eg boxers and labradors. Heart conditions more common in certain breeds – eg King Charles spaniels.

2. Signs of infection

Head region specially important – dental caries and enlarged sub-maxillary glands not always apparent to owner. Encephalitis can originate from any infected site, and relapses can occur if one of these becomes chronic.

3. Signs of laterality	Head-tilt of sudden onset, or circling, is usually indicative of a cerebro-vascular accident. Unequal pupil size indicates either a CVA or a brain tumour. Hemi-paresis of facial muscles, often shown by drooling of saliva or impaired feeding, also points to a CVA or to a tumour.
4. Presence or absence of nystagmus	Usually associated with cerebro-vascular accident.
5. Reflexes	In primary epilepsy, reflexes are normal inter-ictally; also in incidents of cardiac origin. Reflexes may give evidence of laterality, or of widespread depression; the latter can be evidence of space-occupying lesion or of encephalitis.
6. Hypersensitivity of occipital/upper cervical areas	Almost pathognomic of meningitis.
7. Temperature	Pyrexia is indicative of meningitis, but this stage can be very brief and absence of fever does not preclude the existence of cerebral infection.
8. Condition of coat	Generalised loss of coat, particularly if associated with abnormal thirst or appetite, suggests a tumour of the pituitary which may also affect the surrounding brain tissue.
9. Wasting of temporal muscles	Strongly indicative of cerebral tumour.

4 Treatment

There are two aspects to the treatment of a patient with fits: symptomatic therapy for the fits, and radical treatment of the underlying cause. The latter depends essentially on a correct differential diagnosis. The obvious exception to this general plan is the case of primary epilepsy; here, the only useful therapy is symptomatic, but it may be possible to give useful advice about management including future breeding plans if these are important to the owner.

Symptomatic treatment of fits

Importance of continuous administration of anti-convulsants

Veterinary surgeons should spend some time explaining to the owner the principles involved in therapy, because they may not be self-evident to the layman. In the first place it is important to stress that an anti-convulsant must be given regularly, not just at the time of a fit; it is not unusual to find that an owner has a stock of anticonvulsants in his possession and only gives them for a day or two post-ictally because, so far as he can judge, the animal is quite all right at other times. This regime, achieves nothing; moreover, since any sudden drop in anti-convulsant level in a patient's blood may precipitate status epilepticus, it can be positively dangerous.

Owner's part in determination of correct dose and best anti-convulsant

Secondly, the owner's co-operation must be sought if the correct dose is to be determined satisfactorily. The veterinarian must explain that when medication is given by mouth, and the site of action is in the brain, many factors such as absorption and transport affect the result; hence, a certain amount of trial and error is inevitable. Even the selection of the ideal anti-convulsant cannot be forecast with certainty and every patient must be considered as an individual case.

Significance of side-effects of anti-convulsants

The owner should also be warned that the patient may be mildly ataxic when medication begins but this usually wears off after a few days. If it persists, then the dose probably is too large, and the owner should report the matter to the veterinary surgeon. If this situation is not explained to the owner in the first place, it is quite likely that he will decide the medication is making his dog worse – and stop giving it. Other possible side-effects which should be mentioned are increased thirst, and sometimes, increased hunger. Knowledgeable owners may, quite reasonably begin to worry about kidney function if they have not been warned about the thirst. These effects usually decrease after a few weeks. Phenobarbitone occasionally causes hyperkinesis in dogs so that they pace about and cry ceaselessly, and cases have been reported in which phenobarbitone has been thought to cause liver damage. In the majority of such cases liver damage has been the result of dogs being on a second anticonvulsant, and cases of serious liver damage in dogs treated only with phenobarbitone are rare.

Possible causes of treatment failure

It is also advisable to point out to the owner that an anti-convulsant will not, necessarily control the fits completely, because the high dose-rate needed for this would produce severe ataxia; but the medication should reduce the frequency and/or severity of the fits. This warning forestalls the complaint from the owner that the animal is still having fits, despite regular medication.

Importance of keeping records of fits

If owners like keeping records, it is quite helpful to give them record sheets as supplied by Vétoquinol. This will give useful information if kept for a year or so, and will enable the owners to feel that they are collaborating actively in the scheme of treatment (as indeed they are).

Advice on management

Some guidance as to management is also necessary. If the patient has some condition other than primary epilepsy, that must of course be considered, but as far as the fits are concerned, the animal's life style probably need not be drastically changed. Fits normally occur during relaxation so there is no need to curtail exercise. In some instances police dogs and guide dogs for the blind have continued their normal work quite successfully for many years after the development of primary epilepsy.

Problems related to other dogs in the house

The owner can be assured that a fit is unlikely to occur when the animal is out for a walk; it can, however, occur in a car if the animal is used to travelling and relaxes in the car. If other dogs are kept with the affected animal, there is a slight risk that they will attack the patient during a fit; this risk should be explained to the owner, so that he can re-arrange sleeping quarters if necessary, and if he is in the habit of going out and leaving all the dogs loose in the house, he may like to alter his plans, at least until he can see the reaction of the healthy dogs to the epileptic one at the time of a fit.

Precautions to be taken by owner at time of fit and during recovery

There is little that an owner can, or should, do when a dog has a fit except to ensure that it does not damage itself by falling downstairs, or off a high bed, or into a garden pond. If very young children are around, they should be kept away from the patient until it has fully recovered. Dogs and cats do not usually damage themselves in fits and there is little need for human interference; in particular it is as well to assure the ardent first-aider that there is no need to insert a wedge between the teeth, since dogs seldom bite their tongues when fitting.

As the animal recovers and wanders round without full vision, it may be necessary to shut it in a room with as few obstructions in it as possible, until the whole of the brain has recovered its normal activity. This post-ictal period is very variable – sometimes it lasts half an hour or so, and sometimes it is completely absent.

Specific treatment of primary epilepsy

It is not usual to start treatment if a dog is presented when it has only had one fit, unless the owner insists on having something done. It is always possible that the fit is due to poisoning and that there will be no recurrence, or that it is a case of primary epilepsy with long intervals between the fits. It is best to give the owner some idea of the problem and ask him to note further fits on one of the report sheets issued by Vétoquinol. It is important also to explain to the owner that the dog may be on medication for life and to discuss the financial aspect of this situation.

Essential co-operation of owner

If further fits do occur and the veterinarian feels confident that the correct diagnosis is primary epilepsy, then treatment may be necessary. As mentioned in the earlier part of this chapter, it is necessary to seek the owner's co-operation and explain to him the various problems involved and, in particular, the need to continue medication even if the patient has not had a recent fit.

Anti-convulsants commonly used in the UK

Generic Name	Trade Name	Company
Phenobarbitone	Epiphen	Vétoquinol
Potassium bromide		
Diazepam	Valium	Roche

Guide lines for the administration of anti-convulsants:

1. There is no fixed dose rate for any anti-convulsant.

2. The dose on a body-weight basis is usually much higher for dogs than for cats.

3. Medication should be given at least 12-hourly, possibly giving a larger dose at night than in the morning because the majority of fits occur in the early hours of the morning.

4. Any change in medication must be made gradually over a period of 2 – 3 weeks.

5. The following gives some idea of the dose range for dogs, but the needs of each patient must be studied separately if success is to be achieved:

Phenobarbitone (Epiphen)	2 – 8 mg/kg/12hr
Potassium bromide	22 – 30 mg/kg/day
Diazepam (Valium)	0.5 – 2.0 mg/kg/per rectum or i/v

6. There are several special problems with cats and it is never safe to assume thta the guide-lines given for medication for dogs can be applied to cats. **Phenobarbitone at a dose rate of 2-3 mg/kg/day is the most useful anticonvulsant for cats.** Diazepam may also be useful. Cats should always be given a thiamin supplement because many of them live on a restricted diet which can easily lead to avitaminosis B. It is also useful to bear in mind that potassium bromide is a useful sedative for an excited cat (150-600 mg).

7. It is wise to remember that any defect in detoxification or excretion may lead to unduly high blood levels of anti-convulsants. Likewise, any defect in absorption (eg diarrhoea) may reduce the expected level.

8. Anti-convulsants take some time to reach therapeutic levels in the blood (phenobarbitone – 2-3 wk; potassium bromide – 2-3 months).

Many other drugs can be used – in fact any of the drugs listed in the pharmacopoeia for the treatment of Grand Mal in human beings are possible and a number of them have been found to be successful in individual dogs.

Particular mention should be made of potassium bromide. In the early part of this century this drug was widely used in human medicine as an anti-convulsant, but when phenobarbitone was introduced in 1912, potassium bromide was abandoned because of its toxicity. Recently many veterinarians have used potassium bromide as an adjunct to phenobarbitone in difficult cases. Great care should be taken if this regime is adopted as bromism is an insidious and serious form of poisoning. Usage of potassium bromide as a solution can allow more accurate dosing. Combined with regular serum sampling and a constant dietary salt intake it is possible to significantly reduce the risks of bromide toxicity.

Long-term management of medication

It is not desirable to give continuous medication to a dog for a number of years because habituation occurs and because of the danger of liver damage; the ideal scheme is to find a drug and dose which control the fits to an acceptable frequency, and then **gradually** reduce the dose and, hopefully, eventually withdraw it altogether. The dog can then be left without medication until the fits recur at sufficiently short intervals to warrant further therapy; with this regime the dose can be kept low enough to avoid serious side-effects. Many dogs suffering from primary epilepsy live a normal life-span if treated in this way and, finally, die from some other cause.

Prolonged administration of phenobarbitone at high dosage can damage the liver but proven cases are fairly rare. Dual therapy with phenytoin is one of the commonest cause of liver toxicity when using phenobarbitone and this combination should be avoided. It is often possible to keep the phenobarbitone dosage down by giving potassium bromide, which is not metabolised by the liver, with phenobarbitone. There are a number of liver function tests that can be used to assess liver damage but is very important that the right tests are used and that they are interpreted correctly. Those relating to albumin and to bile are the most useful.

Status epilepticus: management and causes

Sometimes, however, the results are less good and may provide either an acute emergency or a chronic problem. The acute emergency is status epilepticus, when the dog has one fit after another for a period of hours; this situation will end fatally if not treated correctly. The dog must immediately be hospitalised, an adequate airway established and the fits controlled with diazepam (Valium); usually this can be achieved with a total dose of 5-25 mg; ideally this is given intravenously but, if this proves impossible, it can be given per rectum; if this drug is not available, phenobarbitone (30-60 mg) can be used. Pentobarbitone sodium (Nembutal) is not satisfactory as the animal frequently goes into convulsions again as the anaesthesia lightens. Intravenous injection to effect is ideal but if this is not possible the drug must be administered by any route available. Cardiac and respiratory function should be monitored and homoeostasis maintained until consciousness returns; hopefully, this will take place without recurrence of convulsions but, if further fits do occur, more sedative must be given.

The most common cause of status epilepticus is sudden cessation of medication, either through oversight, or the owner's failure to appreciate the need for continuous medication with only a gradual decrease, if circumstances warrant it, over an agreed period of time. Provided that the dog is hospitalised reasonably soon after the development of status epilepticus, and that fits do not recur as consciousness returns, the prognosis is fairly good. Many epileptic dogs have just one incident of status epilepticus in their lives, and many of them live for many years after such an incident.

Possible causes of long-term treatment failure.
Significance of increase in fit frequency

The chronic problem is less well understood. Some dogs whose fits have been reasonably controlled with anti-convulsants for years, suddenly seem to become refractory to their effect, and even large doses no longer control the frequency of the fits to any appreciable extent. This situation may be caused by some change in the brain cells, or a decrease in the animal's ability to absorb, or transport, the drug, or some other factor having an adverse effect on cerebral function, such as a cerebral tumour or a head injury.

Sometimes a change of anti-convulsant helps, but often there is no obvious solution and the prognosis is grave. This situation seems to occur more commonly in certain susceptible breeds, but reliable figures are difficult to obtain.

If a dog has a mild toxaemia from some illness unconnected with the central nervous system (eg nephritis), the frequency of fits in an epileptic dog may be increased; this does not necessarily indicate any permanent deterioration in the brain and, if the illness is treated successfully, the fit frequency will, in due course, revert to its former level. It is important to explain this to owners since they will otherwise interpret an increase in fit frequency as a very grave sign.

Most brain lesions, such as tumours, can give rise to a variety of clinical signs, depending on the exact location of the lesion, but it has been shown that if a dog has primary epilepsy, almost any other brain lesion is likely, initially, to produce an increase in fit frequency. Hence, differential diagnosis of the cause of any increase in fit frequency is difficult but very important from the point of view of prognosis.

Before admitting defeat, when an anti-convulsant seems to be losing its effect, it is worth asking the following questions:

1.   Is the animal getting the prescribed daily dose (some tablets only reach the carpet !) ?

2.   Is the dose large enough? Regular blood tests are essential to monitor the amount of anti-convulsant absorbed.

3.   Might a different or additional anti-convulsant be more successful?

4.   Is the diagnosis correct?

Advice for breeders

The veterinary surgeon must be prepared to advise a breeder who is concerned about the heritability of primary epilepsy. In the first place he must be satisfied that the diagnosis has been properly established: assuming this to be so, the most practical advice that the veterinarian can give, in the light of present-day knowledge, is not to breed from the affected animal, and not to mate together again, the dog and bitch which produced the affected animal. Information about litter-mates of an affected animal is helpful and close-breeding should be avoided. If primary epilepsy occurs in a bitch, and if the frequency of the fits seems to be connected in any way with the oestrous cycle, spaying or hormonal control may help considerably in controlling the fits – in fact, in some bitches it seems to effect a cure.

Contra-indications for tranquillisers, whether intended for sedation or pre-medication

It is important to realise that tranquillisers are contra-indicated in primary epilepsy; this follows logically from the fact that fits normally occur when a dog is relaxed or quiescent. This fact has particular relevance in two situations; the first occurs when the owner is alarmed, perhaps because he has to take an epileptic dog on a journey, and begs the veterinary surgeon to provide something "just to keep the dog quiet on the journey", or perhaps while he is away for a week end and leaving his dog in charge of another member of the family. It is difficult for an owner not to associate fits with excitement.

The second situation is when a dog is going to have a general anaesthetic, or perhaps have a minor operation under a local anaesthetic: in either case it may well be standard procedure in the practice to give acetylpromazine or a similar tranquilliser as premedication; this may well precipitate fits in a dog with primary epilepsy.

A similar problem may arise when a dog is transported by plane or ship; tranquillisers are regularly given on these occasions unless precise instructions have been given to the contrary. It is particularly important that a crated animal should not have a fit, since it could easily suffer serious, or even fatal, injury in a confined space of this type.

Complementary medicine

In some dogs good results have been reported from complementary medicine, acupuncture, herbal medicine and homoeopathy in particular. If an owner expresses an interest, the veterinarian should be prepared to refer him/her to a suitably qualified colleague. The alternative treatment is carried out while the patient continues with the orthodox medicine.

Primary epilepsy in other species

It is fairly rare for a veterinary surgeon to be asked to treat primary epilepsy in species other than dogs. However, it has been shown that phenobarbitone can be used for a wide variety of species, including the cat and the horse. Treatment for horses cannot be recommended, because of possible danger to riders, since it is unlikely that fits can be wholly eliminated.

Treatment of underlying causes

The foregoing gives details about treatment of primary epilepsy, but if some other condition has been diagnosed, then in addition to the administration of anti-convulsants consideration must be given to the underlying condition. Notes relevant to the more common of these, follow.

Internal hydrocephalus

The most useful treatment for internal hydrocephalus is a course of a diuretic. The condition can be congenital or acquired; if it is acquired, consideration must be given to the cause and treatment attempted for this as well as for the hydrocephalus. The congenital condition should be treated as early as possible, so that pressure atrophy is eliminated before permanent brain damage occurs. Breeds of dog with domed skulls are more susceptible than others, and it is wise to remember this fact throughout the animal's life; any other brain condition may give rise to hydrocephalus in a susceptible animal, or any condition which affects the water balance of the patient. It is also worth remembering that raised intra-cranial pressure comprises a risk for general anaesthesia; halothane should be avoided and the lowest level of premedication and barbiturate anaesthesia used if surgery is essential.

Meningitis and encephalitis

It is not always possible to identify the causal organism, but investigations have shown that it is more frequently bacterial rather than viral, and therefore it is reasonable to attempt to treat patients with antimicrobials. There is a problem however in that the blood-brain barrier may prevent the medication reaching the organism. In acute meningitis the barrier becomes more permeable, but many animals have chronic encephalitis and the barrier is then a very important factor. The change in permeability of the barrier can be responsible for apparent relapses; when the infection is acute, medication reaches the site and the patient improves – then, as the inflammation is reduced the integrity of the blood-brain barrier increases, medication is less effective and the infection re-appears.

Antibacterials: dosage

The most useful antimicrobials available at the present time:

Trimethoprium-sulphonamide antibacterials

These antibacterials should be given for 5-7 days after cessation of clinical symptoms. They have few side-effects but occasionally folate deficiency occurs, so a supplement of vitamin B should be given. Chloramphenicol should not be used if the dog is having phenobarbitone.

Toxoplasmosis

If there is reason to think that toxoplasma infection is responsible for the encephalitis, Clindamycin (ll mg/kg/day up to 28 days), may be helpful in addition to the foregoing.

Head injury

In the case of head injury treatment depends on the time that has elapsed since the injury was inflicted. If the accident has occurred 72 hours or less before the veterinarian sees the patient, the likelihood of fits as a long-term complication can be greatly reduced by appropriate therapy. This consists of a diuretic together with phenobarbitone. Experimental work in human medicine has shown that much of the permanent brain damage from a head injury is due to the development of cerebral oedema, and that this can be successfully counteracted by diuretics. The use of sedatives as soon after the injury as possible, without waiting to see if fits will appear, has been shown to have a big influence on the likelihood of later development of fits. The duration of the treatment should be several weeks, depending on the patient's progress, and the severity of the original injury.

If the accident has occurred months, or even years, earlier, the situation is often described as "secondary epilepsy", and in this case, treatment is identical with that for primary epilepsy.

Cerebro-vascular accidents

Cerebro-vascular accidents occur in adult cats, dogs and horses of all ages; they do become somewhat more frequent after middle age, but many younger animals sustain them, too. There is little that can be done about the cerebro-vascular accident which has already occurred, since it is not possible to know whether the accident is basically due to clotting or bleeding. Animals often make fairly good recoveries from cerebro-vascular accidents, except when special senses are involved, but treatment must be directed towards prevention of further similar accidents. Cardiac dysfunction can be involved, and this possibility must be checked, together with prothrombin time, haemoglobin level, and other blood characteristics. The possibility of warfarin poisoning must be borne in mind, if prothrombin time is extended.

Space-occupying lesion

If the lesion is an abscess, it is possible that it can be reduced by administration of an antibiotic; if it is a cyst or haematoma, the clinical effects may decrease with time and all that needs to be done is to treat the signs (fits) with an anti-convulsant. If, on the other hand, the clinical picture points to a tumour, there is usually no effective treatment. Strangely, in such cases, corticosteroids sometimes produce a dramatic remission for a few weeks, but subsequently the patient usually deteriorates rapidly. Occasionally, if the tumour is circumscribed and on the sufface of the brain, surgery may be possible. An MRI scan would be an essential preliminary.

Poisoning

If fits occur as the result of recent ingestion of poison, the situation is similar to that described under status epilepticus. In the first instance diazepam (Valium) should be given to control the convulsions. The patient should then be hospitalised and placed under continuous observation. Steps to identify the poison and, if possible, administer an antidote can then be taken.

The detailed treatment of poisoning is beyond the scope of this book, but a few points may usefully be stressed. If an animal is convulsing, nothing must be given by mouth and no attempt made to induce emesis until the convulsions have been controlled.

Strychnine

Pentobarbitone sodium can be used to control the convulsions caused by strychnine but it is important to remember to monitor the patient continuously because hyperactivity of the nervous system can be converted easily to irreversible respiratory depression.

Metaldehyde

Fits resulting from ingestion of "meta" are usually accompanied by extensive muscular tremors; these tremors are not set off by external stimuli as are those of strychnine poisoning. Some dogs develop a liking for "meta" and care must be taken to prevent repetition of the mishap.

Lead

Sources of lead are very varied and include linoleum, golf balls, old paint and plastic toys. Gastric signs usually precede those of the central nervous system and, hence, lead poisoning can mimic the effects of canine distemper. The fits associated with lead poisoning are due to cerebral oedema, so it is in order to give mannitol or a corticosteroid as well as an anti-convulsant. As with strychnine, it is easy to overdose with a sedative. It is not unusual for a relapse to occur after an animal has been successfully treated for plumbism, particularly if it exerts itself, so convalescence is essential. Plumbism is rare in cats as they are fastidious feeders.

Warfarin

If a poison based on warfarin has been ingested, then the onset of fits may be delayed for a long time; the cause of the fits is usually pressure from a haematoma in the brain but this will probably form very slowly. In such cases, vitamin K, together with an anti-convulsant is the best line of therapy.

5 Prognosis

An informed prognosis must depend, in the first place, on a correct diagnosis; even then, the outcome of any condition involving the central nervous system of a living animal, is uncertain. However, the veterinarian is often pressed to give some opinion, and he can but draw upon his own knowledge and experience, and upon that of others whom he trusts, and explain the position to his client as lucidly as possible. He must also bear in mind that his opinion may be of interest to the insurers of the animal in question, and it is therefore necessary to be very careful in forecasts of the animal's future usefulness, and of the aetiology of the illness and of its hereditary significance.

Primary epilepsy

An increased tendency to have fits is part of the epileptic animal's make-up, and this will not be affected by any treatment. Some control of fit-frequency can usually be achieved by long-term administration of anti-convulsants and, in some bitches, spaying or hormonal control produces a marked improvement. The condition does not itself become more serious with age, although any general deterioration in health, such as chronic nephritis, will tend to increase fit-frequency. It must also be admitted that in a few animals habituation to the usual anti-convulsants occurs and ever-increasing dosage is needed to control the fits, and this may produce an intolerable situation for both client and patient.

Animals suffering from primary epilepsy do not normally die from this condition, and it does not appear to shorten the life-span of the individual. Owners often worry that the heart will be damaged by the apparent violence of the heart-beat during and after a fit, but there is no evidence to support this fear.

Congenital hydrocephalus

In congenital hydrocephalus the prognosis is affected partly by the severity and partly by the time for which the condition has been in existence before treatment. If the skull is obviously more domed than would be natural for the breed, and if an open fontanelle can be palpated, the hydrocephalus is probably severe and the prognosis poor.

Again, if the animal has shown clinical signs for weeks or months, it is probable that pressure atrophy will have caused irreversible brain damage. If, on the other hand, there is no obvious anatomical abnormality, and signs have been slight, or only occasionally present, and the animal is still growing, the prognosis is good. There will always be a risk of recurrence, but treatment should resolve further incidents, particularly if the owner (or the animal's record card) is able to provide evidence of the earlier condition, so that differential diagnosis is facilitated.

Acquired internal hydrocephalus

Acquired internal hydrocephalus is always secondary to some other illness which has caused a disturbance in the water balance, or to cerebral trauma or infection leading to oedema of the brain cells. Providing that the basic cause can be treated successfully, acquired hydrocephalus can often be resolved without leaving any permanent brain damage.

Meningitis and encephalitis

It is very difficult to make any reliable prediction about meningitis and encephalitis unless the nature of the infecting organism is known, together with its sensitivity to antibiotics. This may occasionally be possible in an epidemic, or when a post-mortem examination has been carried out on an in-contact animal.

The acute form of meningitis can often be treated successfully, provided therapy is started soon enough and facilities for nursing a very ill patient are available. It is important to explain to the owner that the antibiotic will, hopefully, eliminate the organism concerned, but there is still a need for the animal to repair damaged brain cells and this will take time, so fits may occur for some weeks after termination of antibiotic therapy. In general, if a patient does not die from acute meningitis, it recovers completely.

A different problem arises when the infection is chronic and less severe. In such cases the signs frequently abate during antibiotic therapy, only to flare up as soon as treatment ends. Sometimes, an extra-cerebral focus of infection exists (eg ears, sinus, tonsil etc) and if this can be eliminated, perhaps by surgery or by local treatment, complete recovery results. If, however, the persistent infection seems confined to the brain, and fits become frequent whenever antibiotic therapy ceases, euthanasia may be the only sensible course.

Head injury

Most animals make surprisingly good recoveries from accidents involving head injuries, provided that cerebral oedema has not been severe or long-lasting. If an animal has sustained concussion and is being nursed in an intensive care unit, it should be possible to establish a reasonably reliable prognosis with assistance from radiography and electro-encephalography; this is one of the few occasions when an EEG gives valuable information that cannot be deduced by any other means.

Head injuries do often lead to scar formation on the brain, and such scars provide irritant foci, which in turn give rise to fits. This secondary or symptomatic epilepsy tends to diminish with time, so the prognosis for this aspect of a head injury is not too serious.

Legal complications may ensue if there is any question of compensation for the damage from the head injury; the scar may not form for some months after the accident and this means that the occurrence of fits may not be connected in the owner's mind with the original accident.

Cerebro-vascular disease

Prognosis from an isolated cerebro-vascular accident is good, unless the sight has been affected; complete restoration of sight is rare. If there is generalised cerebro-vascular disease as a result of ageing, the process can be slowed by appropriate treatment, but not reversed. Cats, in particular, respond well to therapy.

It is important to realise that a cerebro-vascular accident may be secondary to the growth of a brain tumour, or to warfarin poisoning; in these cases the prognosis is obviously less good.

Space occupying lesions

The prognosis for an animal with a tumour affecting the activity of the brain is virtually hopeless at the present time; the lesion is seldom on the surface of the brain, so surgery is not feasible. It must also be remembered that a brain tumour is often a secondary growth, so excision does not really provide an effective cure.

Poisoning

The prognosis for poisoning cannot really be generalised, since it depends on so many variables: the nature of the poison, the quantity ingested, the interval between ingestion and initiation of therapy, the age and condition of the patient, and so on. In general, it can be said that if the patient survives the initial onset of fits, and an effective antidote can be given, there will be no lasting brain damage.

6 Problems

Psychology of the owner

The majority of owners are genuinely terrified when first they see an animal in a fit; they experience a very primitive fear, possibly associated with stories of rabies, and often expect their pets to attack them as soon as they are able to get to their feet. An owner may telephone his veterinary surgeon at this stage, and it is essential that whoever normally takes calls in the practitioner's absence (secretary, receptionist, nurse, spouse) knows how to reassure such a client. Apart from explaining that the animal has not "gone mad", it is useful to warn the owner that, when the patient does get to its feet, it may pace about for some time and blunder into furniture, but this does not mean that it is permanently blind – it is just that the part of the brain concerned with vision is one of the last parts to return to full activity.

Factors affecting management of dog with primary epilepsy

The advisability of keeping a dog or cat with primary epilepsy alive must be considered in the context of the normal life of the whole household. Fits are likely to occur when the animal is relaxed and at home, if the owner goes out frequently, leaving someone else alone with the pet, thought must be given as to whether they will understand and be able to cope with the emergency. In particular, children and elderly persons may have untoward experiences.

There is also the potential danger of the patient being attacked by other animals while in a fit, with possibly fatal results if someone is not on hand to separate them. Usually other animals ignore an animal having a fit, but it is not wise to rely on this, since occasional fatalities have been recorded.

First aid for dog having a fit

It is wise to warn an owner that an animal's temper may be unreliable when it first rises after a fit and before it has fully regained consciousness; people have been bitten in this situation by animals which would never do such a thing if fully conscious. It is also helpful to re-assure owners that there is no need to insert a piece of wood between the teeth of an animal in a fit; it is unlikely that it will bite its tongue, and even if it does, the injury is usually not severe. The only first aid necessary is to move it from the edge of a pond, or the top of a flight of stairs, or the proximity of an open fire, and this can be done by throwing a blanket or coat over it first and then gathering it up, or if afraid even to do that, pushing the covered animal with the foot.

Long-term management of primary epilepsy

Once the owner has survived the horror of the first fit, advice on management for the future must be given; this requires, at least a putative, differential diagnosis. If the animal is thought to have primary epilepsy, it is important to stress that it is not ill and need not be cossetted, nor need normal activity be restricted; the fits will occur during periods of relaxation or sleep, **not** when the animal is excited or overactive. It is perhaps worth instancing, in this connection, that there have been Olympic athletes who were epileptic, and they were able to train and perform successfully without fear of fits. Working dogs can continue to work satisfactorily with primary epilepsy, and there are a number of guide dogs and Police Dogs in this category. This information helps clients to appreciate that primary epilepsy does not affect intelligence.

Management of horse with primary epilepsy

Fits in horses are a little less predictable; the consequence for the human partner would be serious if the horse had a fit while working. There have, in fact, been epileptic equines which have performed successfully on the race-course and in the show-ring, but it would be unwise for a veterinary surgeon to recommend a client to continue riding a horse known to have primary epilepsy.

Need for regular medication

The most common problem with treatment is the need to convince the owner that medication must be continued, even though the animal has not had a fit for a few days – or even a few weeks; there is a natural tendency for an owner to consider that the animal is cured, and drop the medication between one day and the next. Admittedly, the veterinarian is probably planning to reduce, and then discontinue, the medication if all goes well, but it is essential that the whole regime, is planned by him, with the intelligent co-operation of the owner. The veterinarian should assess the extent to which his client can understand the rationale of treatment, and hence take an active part in the planning, and explain what is to be done accordingly.

Another common problem is that clients think that their supply of anti-convulsants is only to be used if the animal has a fit; they force down a tablet or capsule immediately **after** the animal has had a fit, having given virtually no medication since the previous fit which may have been some months before.

Tailoring dose

There are several problems related to the patient itself; in particular the fact that there is no rule of thumb for calculation of dosage, and no way of knowing which is the best anti-convulsant for any particular animal. The aim must always be to find the anti-convulsant which controls the fits well, at a dose-rate which causes minimal side-effects. Bodyweight can provide a guide for an initial dose-rate, but one must be prepared to halve or double this, according to the clinical response. This variation from one individual to another is due to pharmacokinetic factors: the drug is administered orally but its site of action is the brain, and there are many different factors influencing absorption, metabolism and excretion. Blood tests by which the effective level of anti-convulsant can be determined should be done at regular intervals so that the ideal dosage can be arranged for each patient.

Clinical history

Since the patient is often normal in appearance by the time that the veterinary surgeon sees it, much reliance must be placed on the owner's observations. There are several pitfalls here: the first is the question of unconsciousness – most people equate this with flaccidity and hence assert that a pet in the tonic and clonic stages of a fit is **not** unconscious. It is perhaps better to ask if the animal seems "disorientated" or "unconnected with its surroundings". A second pitfall arises from the fact that owners may not have seen the beginning of the fit; they may come home and find the dog pacing round and round the room bumping into the furniture and then they may just describe this to the veterinary surgeon. If behaviour which could be a late stage of an epileptic fit is described, it is wise to inquire whether the preceding activity of the animal was known – and whether it might have been a fit. Differential diagnosis between primary epilepsy and a cerebro-vascular accident may otherwise present a problem.

Future management

When the future of an animal with primary epilepsy is being considered, it is vital to try to convince the owner that the somewhat grotesque appearance of a convulsing animal is not an expression of pain. Evidence for this view is derived from human beings with the same condition, from the EEG, and from the fact that the animal will cheerfully lie down in the same place the next day, and so obviously has no untoward memory of the fit.

Heredity

Hereditary factors play some part in determining a tendency to primary epilepsy; it is generally believed that the mode of inheritance is polygenic, and result from either to recessive genes, or to dominant genes with incomplete penetrance. It also appears that there is slight sex linkage making the condition a little more common in male dogs than in bitches. It has been calculated that it would take a 10-year study of 1,000 dogs to investigate fully the mode of inheritance !

If a practitioner is called to diagnose the cause of fits in a dog which has parents or close relatives known to suffer epilepsy, it is certainly sensible to consider primary epilepsy as a possible cause. However, it is essential to remember that reliable diagnosis of a related animal's fits may not have been obtained; rumour often runs wild once a dog has had a fit. Sometimes a dog is said to have "epilepsy", and related dogs are suspected, and then it is found that the original dog had a fit as a result of a road traffic accident with a head injury.

On the other hand, many breeders will affirm that there is no epilepsy in their lines when they are not really in a position to know; the fits of primary epilepsy commonly occur when dogs are asleep, and if the dogs are kennelled at night, nobody may know about the fits. There is also the point that the first fit in primary epilepsy does not usually occur until the dog is over a year old, and many breeders may not ever know that puppies which they have sold, have later developed primary epilepsy. Allowances must be made for reluctance on the part of breeders to reveal facts which may prejudice their reputation. Finally, since there is no bar to showing or working a dog with primary epilepsy, it is quite possible for champions to have this condition.

Conclusion

The treatment and management of dogs with epilepsy can never be simple. It requires the expert knowledge of the veterinary surgeon, together with the understanding, common sense and vigilance of the owner. If all the members of the team, veterinary surgeons, nurses, technicians, owners and breeders co-operate and play their part, there is no reason why many dogs with epilepsy should not lead long, active and happy lives.

Glossary

Adenitis	Inflammation of a gland
Aetiology	Cause (of disease or condition)
Anoxia	Shortage of oxygen
Anticonvulsants	Medicines used to control convulsions
Ataxia	Impaired control of movement
Atrophy	Wasting of tissue
Aura	Warning or premonition of impending attack or fit
Avitaminosis	Lack of vitamin
Cerebral anoxia	Lack of oxygen supply to the brain
Cerebral oedema	Accumulation of fluid in the brain
Cerebro-vascular	Relating to the blood supply of the brain
Chorea(-ic)	Twitching of muscle groups
Clonus(-ic)	Regular alternating contraction and relaxation of muscles (of limbs)
Congenital abnormality	An abnormality which occurs in the uterus and is present at birth
Conjunctivitis	Inflammation of the eyelids
Differential diagnosis	Study of different possible causes of signs
Electro-cardiography	Measurement of the electric pulses from the heart
Electro-encephalography	Measurement of the electric pulses from the brain
Encephalitis	Inflammation of the brain
Encephalopathy	Degeneration of the brain
Epileptogenic	Giving rise to epilepsy
Fontanelle	Junction of several bones of skull on top of head
Haematoma(-ta)	Localised mass of blood outside blood vessel (may be clotted)
Haemoglobin	Red pigment in the blood which carries oxygen
Hemiparesis	Partial paralysis of one side
Hyperglycaemia	Increased amount of sugar in the blood
Hyperkinesis	Excessive activity
Hypoglycaemia	Reduced amount of sugar in the blood

Idiopathic	Having no apparent cause
Inter-ictal	Between convulsions
Internal hydrocephalus	Excess fluid within the skull, pressing on the brain
Interstitial nephritis	Inflammation of the kidney
MRI	Magnetic Resonance Imaging giving picture of internal organs
Meningitis	Inflammation of the membrane covering the brain
Neoplasia	Tumour
Neuron	Nerve cell
Nystagmus	Abnormal, jerky, to-and-fro movement of the eyes
Oestrus	Season (heat), period of sexual interest in female animal
Ophthalmoscopy	Examination of the eye with instruments
Pathognomonic	Applied to sign characteristic of a particular disease or condition
Pathology	Abnormal change in part of the body
Pharmacokinetic	Relating to movement of drugs in the body
Photophobia	Dislike of light
Post-ictal	After convulsion
Prothrombin time	Indication of time taken for blood to clot
Protozoal infection	Infection with a protozoa
Pyrexia	Raised body temperature
Status epilepticus	Condition in which fits follow each other very quickly for a long period of time
Tonic	Relating to a state of continuous muscular contraction
Torticollis	Twisted neck
Toxaemia	Presence of poisons in the blood stream
Vermifuge	Agent intended to remove parasitic intestinal worms
Water-loading	Tending to increase fluid content of body

Patient's Record

Name of animal

Breed

Sex   Date of birth

Dates "on heat"

Details of fits

Date	Time of day or night	Place (indoors/outside)	Medication	Interval since last fit